Strong Body for Athletes

A 30-day step-by-step guide to losing weight and improve your body with a high-protein diet plan. Strong muscles and a healthy brain in a perfect body.

Katia Kolner

Test of Contents

Introduction

Vegan athletes need to be aware of what they eat and how much they eat to absorb the required nutrition that supports muscle function, repair, endurance, strength, and motivation as these are qualities that professional athletes' treasure. Protein features high on the list of what to eat. You should also consider your calorie intake, macro and micro nutritional sources and amino acids, some of which may need to be supplemented. Proteins and carbohydrates average at four calories per gram, while fats average at nine calories per gram. Following this, it is possible to calculate how much of each nutrient type to consume per day.

When planning your vegan diet, an athlete may need to consider their exercise routines, as those who gym may have high impact days (such as the dreaded "leg-day") and lower impact days where their bodies need more nutrients geared at repair work. For every athlete, their meal plans will be uniquely based on their age, weight, level of activity, food availability (veggies and fruits tend to be seasonal), and personal taste. You certainly don't have to eat buckets of beans to be a vegan.

Converting to the vegan diet from an omnivore diet may, surprisingly, be a huge mental shock; however, there are some changes to your digestive system to consider as well. Vegans consume more dietary fiber than most omnivores, hence, your gut may go through stages of feeling somewhat bloated. You will need to consume more water as well. There are many suggested ratios, yet the easiest is to work per calorie. A fast rule of 1 milliliter water per calorie seems easy enough to follow. Keeping in mind that the volume of your food may increase, you may also need to eat quite a while earlier than an omnivore would before exercising. So, the usual rule of an hour fast before eating may need to be extended to 90 minutes fast before exercising.

Always consider adding variety to your vegan diet as this increases the opportunity for your body to consume all of the vital amino acids, and this leads to better protein synthesis (which is essential for developing muscle tone and recovering from injuries). Plant-based meals are very filling due to their high fiber content, yet you need to consume a larger amount to meet your calorie requirements. To avoid feeling too sated, you can gain extra carbs from eating nuts and seeds throughout the day as snacks.

Finally, when adding the finishing touches to your training program, it is essential that you intersperse training sessions with sufficient time to ensure that your muscles have time to rest and recover (where you rebuild their energy reserves, hydrate your body, and restore the normal chemical balance of your metabolism). Short-term rest periods may be anything from taking a few minutes break before moving on to the next training activity or even taking the rest of the day off after a particularly strenuous session. Professional athletes know that the body may be a machine, but it is a machine that needs to have "down time" too. It would be best to do a training log where you record what you have eaten, how long you fasted before training, and how you felt during and after the training session. This will also help you to assess whether you need to add more carbs or proteins to your diet, and if you require a longer rest period before moving on to the next training activity.

If you struggle with fatigue (or the shakes) after strenuous activities, you may need to increase your amino acid consumption or get more zinc and iron into your system. Basically, we are all unique, and what works for another vegan athlete may not work for you. This training log can also allow you to experiment with perhaps moving to shorter training sessions with more frequent rest periods to achieve the same level of fitness and muscle building. No two professional athletes train the same way. Listen to your body and your gut to find a way that works for you.

Lastly, don't forget to get enough sleep. Mental fatigue can easily translate as physical symptoms. Insomnia may also be caused by a deficiency in magnesium. This could be caused by strenuous activity that consumes natural minerals in the body. Taking a magnesium supplement or eating some dark chocolate or half a banana before sleep can help create restful sleep.

Fortunately, the Internet allows for the development of support networks for vegan athletes. What we eat says a lot about us, and vegans can be successful, high-achieving athletes with planning and experimentation to find what works for their unique body.

Tips in Starting Plant-Based Diet
Plan your Weight Loss

1. Make a list of 15-20 of your favorite foods

To make this list, sit down with your whole family and ask everyone about their favorite foods. Once this is done, look at the list and select those foods that are easy and quick to prepare and do not need too many ingredients.

The best if they are healthy meals.

2. Gather the recipes of the meals you are going to prepare

Organize your list. You can divide the meals into groups, for example: soups, meat dishes, vegetarian dishes and so on, so that it is easy to handle them.

Find the recipes you need and write them down or print them on sheets of paper. Also, you may consider buying a special notebook for recipes. The most important thing is to have easy access to them, because you will need them often.

3. Plan all-day meals

Don't just create a list of lunches. It is advisable to eat 3-5 times a day, so think about planning all breakfasts, lunches and dinners.

This will avoid eating out, it will help you plan and use your cooking time better. You will also have the opportunity to make better use of food leftovers (it is important if you want to maximize the savings effect).

4. Write your menu on paper

You have many ways to do it. You can use a notebook. On the other side you write a list of your meals, and on the right write all the necessary ingredients to prepare this meal (at one time you will have a meal plan and the shopping list).

Regardless of which method you choose, put your plan in a place clearly visible to all members of the house. The best place is the kitchen.

5. Check what you have in your pantry

Before putting your menu into action, it is a good idea to check your pantry, refrigerator and freezer first. Organize all the food you have there: throw away what is already expired, and order everything else in appropriate groups (go to the shopping list template to see an example of groups)

Plan meals based on the products you already have. For example, do you have pasta? Write pasta on your food list for the next day. If you like chicken pasta, but you don't have it, then write "chicken" on your shopping list.

In this way, you will reduce the supermarket account and also avoid unnecessary purchases of products that you already have at home. In addition, it is the first step to keep your refrigerator and pantry in order.

6. Adjust the menu according to your family's eventualities

When you are planning meals, consider your daily activities and those of your family. Did your children eat lunch at school? That day plan a more modest lunch at home. Do you come back late from work? Think of a dinner that takes little time to prepare. Has the family been invited to a Sunday dinner? You don't have to prepare dinner that day.

It is good to consider all the related factors and take them into account when creating your menu.

7. Use the seasonal products

Depending on the season, the availability of individual fruits and vegetables can change dramatically. Therefore, their prices also change. The best prices will be found during the harvest, which becomes savings.

The point is that it is normal that your menu can change during the year.

I recommend using fresh ingredients from your garden season or those that are available in the market this season.

8. Prepare more meals at once

Do you consider eating the same dish more than once in the week? Try to prepare a larger amount of this meal, for today and the next few days. If you do, put the food separately in containers and place them in the refrigerator or freezer, you can also bottle the food in jars.

Another example: for lunch you make chicken breast chops, and you also like salad with chicken breast. Cook more chicken breasts at a time and then store a part in the refrigerator. As a result, in the afternoon or the next day you will prepare your salad much faster.

9. Plan your food cleaning day

If ever by the end of the week you collect all the leftovers from your refrigerator, you can plan a night, when together with your family you will have dinner only leftovers.

That day you should also check which products are near the expiration date and these are the products to use in the meals of the next days. This way you reduce food waste and save money.

10. Review your daily plan

Your meal plan must be flexible. If necessary, don't be afraid to make modifications and use the opportunities.

Many people consider themselves choosy in food before switching to a plant-based diet. However, then they find food for themselves, which they could not even think of. Beans, tofu, different types of sweets from plants - such a meal for a meat lover seems tasteless. So, try a new dish and let your taste buds decide for themselves what they like best.

The 5 Determining Factors for Being Fit

It's is not easy to make a change in any diet that you quickly embrace. The decision to take on a plant-based meal plan is based on wanting to live healthier lives. The change might be inevitable later on after many realizations of what we get when we eventually abandon what we prefer to consume.

1. The first tip is all about setting rules and making sure that you are being initiated to new recipes of plant-based meals even twice a week. Regulations created by yourself will be quickly followed as compared to the ones formed and forced on you. In this plant-based diet, it is all about loving what you are doing. The created recipes will always be easy to follow, and once mastered, you will only be improving on them. One rule that can be created here is the setting of a day. This day is preserved mainly for one purpose, and that's making a plant-based meal. Make it to the family and get their ultimate reviews on what you have done. Ask them to comment on the tastes and the food in general. The result will help you a lot, especially in your next meal.

2. The next tip here is all about creating a constant tendency towards plant-based meals. Make a plan for cooking this food more often within a week. Don't wait for ages to pass since you are getting induced to starting your plant-based diet. Practice makes perfect, and within a long time, your skills, especially necessary skills, will improve. Your experience will be a notch higher, and this will be reflected

in your habits. Making cooking of plant meals frequent is one of the most excellent tips in jump-starting your plant-based meal. Along the way, you will get adapted to it. You'll also realize that you've changed your approach to how you always think of other types of food, such as diets full of meat and junk foods.

3. As a beginner in this diet, the best tip for starting a plant-based diet meal plan will be, to begin with, vegetables. Try your best to eat vegetables. The act can be during lunch and dinner or rather a supper. Ensure that your plate is always full of plants of different categories. Different colors can help you choose the different types you want to get to learn. Vegetables too can also be eaten as snacks, especially when combined with hummus or salsa. You can also use guacamole too in this combination and rest assured you will love it.

4. One tip that will help you in starting a plant-based diet meal is by using whole grains during breakfast. Use it in high quantities since it will help you in adopting this kind of diet within a short period. It is not always easy to use all of these whole grains. The best way forward is to choose meals that can suit you and the rest of your family at first. Good examples will be highly recommended. These might include oats, barley, or even buckwheat. Here, you can add some flavors provided by different types of nuts and several seeds. Don't forget to include fresh fruits next to your reach.

5. Another tip is about pairing foods. You can use this tool to have more excellent knowledge of which types of plant-based foods can be matched and results in good taste. You can do this pairing by combining several flavors. The result should give you a strong feeling that works for you.

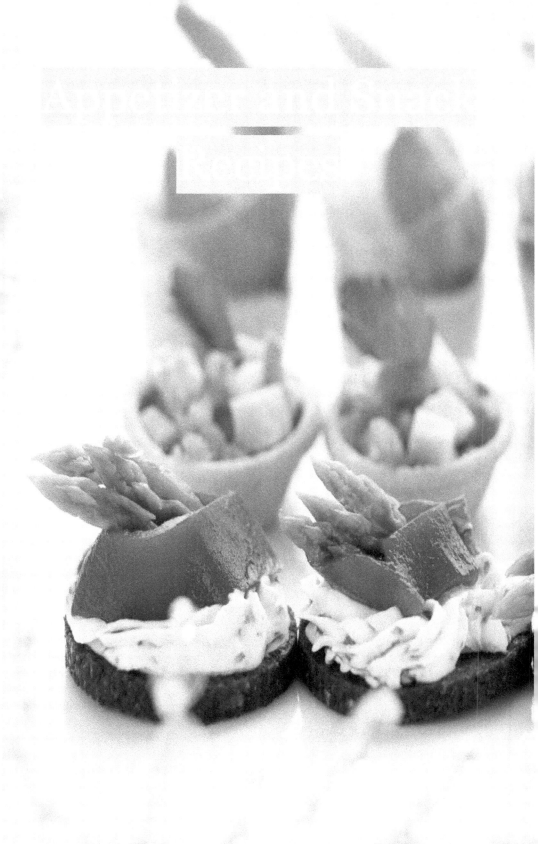

1. The Garbanzo Bean Extravaganza

Preparation Time: 10 minutes

Cooking Time: 0 minute

Servings: 5

Ingredients:

- 1 can garbanzo beans, chickpeas
- 1 tablespoon olive oil
- 1 teaspoon sunflower seeds
- 1 teaspoon garlic powder
- ½ teaspoon paprika

Directions:

1. Preheat your oven to 375 degrees Fahrenheit
2. In baking sheet line with silicone baking mat
3. Drain and rinse garbanzo beans, pat garbanzo beans dry and put into a large bowl
4. Toss with olive oil, sunflower seeds, garlic powder, paprika and mix well
5. Spread over a baking sheet
6. Cook for 20 minutes at 190 Celsius
7. Turn chickpeas so they are roasted well
8. Return in the oven for 25 minutes at 375 190 C

9. Let them cool and enjoy!

Nutrition:

395 Calories

52g Carbohydrates

35g Protein

1. Roasted Onions and Green Beans

Preparation Time: 10 minutes

Cooking Time: 15 minutes

Servings: 6

Ingredients:

- 1 yellow onion, sliced into rings
- ½ teaspoon onion powder
- 2 tablespoons coconut flour
- 1 and 1/3 pounds fresh green beans, trimmed and chopped

Directions:

1. Take a large bowl and mix sunflower seeds with onion powder and coconut flour
2. Add onion rings
3. Mix well to coat
4. Spread the rings on the baking sheet, lined with parchment paper
5. Drizzled with some oil
6. Bake for 10 minutes at 400 Fahrenheit
7. Parboil the green beans for 3 to 5 minutes in the boiling water
8. Drain and serve the beans with baked onion rings

9. Eat warm and enjoy!

Nutrition:

214 Calories

3.7g Carbohydrates

8.3g Protein

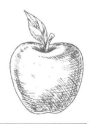

2. Lemony Sprouts

Preparation Time: 11 minutes

Cooking Time: 0 minute

Servings: 3

Ingredients:

- 1-pound Brussels
- 8 tablespoons olive oil
- 1 lemon juice
- ¾ cup spicy almond and seed mix

Directions:

1. Take a bowl and mix in lemon juice, salt, pepper and olive oil
2. Mix well
3. Stir in shredded Brussels and toss
4. Let it sit for 10 minutes
5. Add nuts and toss
6. Serve and enjoy!

Nutrition:

382 Calories

9g Carbohydrates

7g Protein

3. Hummus without Oil

Preparation Time: 5 minutes

Cooking Time: 0 minute

Serving: 6

Ingredients

- 2 tablespoons lemon juice

- 1 15-ounce can chickpeas

- 2 tablespoons tahini

- 2 garlic cloves

- Red pepper hummus

- 2 tablespoons of almond milk pepper

Direction:

1. Cleanse chickpeas and process them in a high-speed blender with garlic until break into fine pieces.

2. Add the other ingredients and blend everything. Add some water if you want a less thick consistency.

Nutrition:

202 calories

35g Carbohydrates

11g Protein

4. Tempting Quinoa Tabbouleh

Preparation Time: 10 minutes

Cooking Time: 10 minutes

Servings: 6

Ingredients

- 1 cup quinoa
- 1 garlic clove
- ½ teaspoon salt
- ½ cup of extra virgin olive oil
- 2 tablespoons lemon juice
- 2 Persian cucumbers
- 2 scallions
- 1-pint cherry tomatoes
- ½ cup fresh mint
- 2/3 cup parsley

Instructions:

1. Boil the quinoa over high heat mixed with salt in 1 ¼ cups of water. Adjust heat to medium-low, then simmer for 10 minutes. Remove and rest for 5 minutes. Fluff it with a fork.

2. Whisk the garlic with the lemon juice. Add the olive oil gradually. Season.

3. On a baking sheet, spread the quinoa and set aside. Mix ¼ of the dressing.

4. Add the tomatoes, scallions, herbs, and cucumber. Toss and season. Add the remaining dressing.

Nutrition:

292 calories

20g Fat

5g Protein

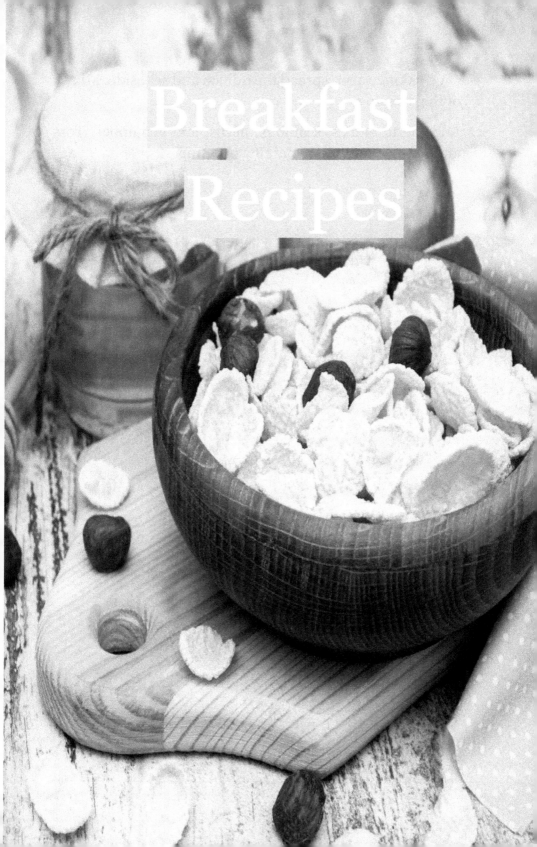

Breakfast
Recipes

5. Chocolate Zoats

Preparation Time: 3 minutes

Cooking Time: 15 minutes

Serving: 1

Ingredient:

- ½ cup rolled oats
- ¾ cup water
- ½ small zucchini, grated (about ½ cup)
- 2 tablespoons powdered chocolate peanut butter

Direction:

1. In a small saucepan bring oats, water, and zucchini to a boil. Cook for 14 minutes. Stir in the powdered peanut butter until it's evenly mixed.

Nutrition:

249 Calories

6g Fat

16g Protein

6. Greens on Toast with Tofu Ricotta

Preparation Time: 5 minutes

Cooking Time: 15 minutes

Serving: 1

Ingredient:

- 2 slices Ezekiel bread
- 1 tablespoon olive oil
- 2 garlic cloves
- 4 cups greens, your choice
- Juice of ½ lemon
- Tofu Ricotta

Direction

1. Toast the Ezekiel bread or English muffin. Meanwhile, warm the oil in a small sauté pan over medium heat. Cook garlic. Mix greens and lemon juice and cook 3 minutes or until the greens are nicely wilted. Season with salt and pepper.

2. Spread about 2 tablespoons of tofu ricotta on each slice of toast, and then top with even amounts of greens. Crack a bit of pepper over them if desired and enjoy right away.

Nutrition:

491 Calories

20g Fat

23g Protein

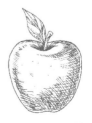

7. Staple Smoothie

Preparation Time: 5 minutes

Cooking Time: 0 minute

Serving: 1

Ingredient:

- 1 (1-ounce) scoop protein powder
- 1 teaspoon-size piece fresh ginger
- 1 teaspoon-size piece fresh turmeric
- 1 cup frozen spinach
- ½ cup frozen blueberries
- 1 teaspoon spirulina
- 1¼ cups water

Direction:

1. Blend all ingredients and process on high speed until smooth.

Nutrition:

185 Calories

3g Fat

28g Protein

8. Cashew Cheese Spread

Preparation Time: 5 minutes

Cooking Time: 0 minute

Serving: 5

Ingredients:

- 1 cup of water
- 1 cup raw cashews
- 1 tsp. nutritional yeast
- ½ tsp. salt
- Optional: 1 tsp. garlic powder

Directions:

1. Immerge the cashews for 6 hours in water.
2. Drain and transfer the soaked cashews to a food processor.
3. Add 1 cup of water and all the other ingredients and blend.

Nutrition:

151 Calories

10.9g Fat

4.6g Protein.

9. Fruit and Nut Oatmeal

Preparation Time: 6 minutes

Cooking Time: 11 minutes

Serving: 2

Ingredients

- ¾ cup rolled oats

- ¼ cup berries, fresh

- ½ ripe banana

- 2 tablespoons nuts

- ½ teaspoon cinnamon

Directions:

1. Position oats in a medium saucepan and add 1½ cups of water. Stir and over high heat, boil. Decrease heat and cook for 5 minutes.

2. Stir in the cinnamon and add the pinch of salt. Serve in 2 bowls and top each with the chopped fruit and nuts.

Nutrition:

420 Calories

21.5g Fat

14 Protein

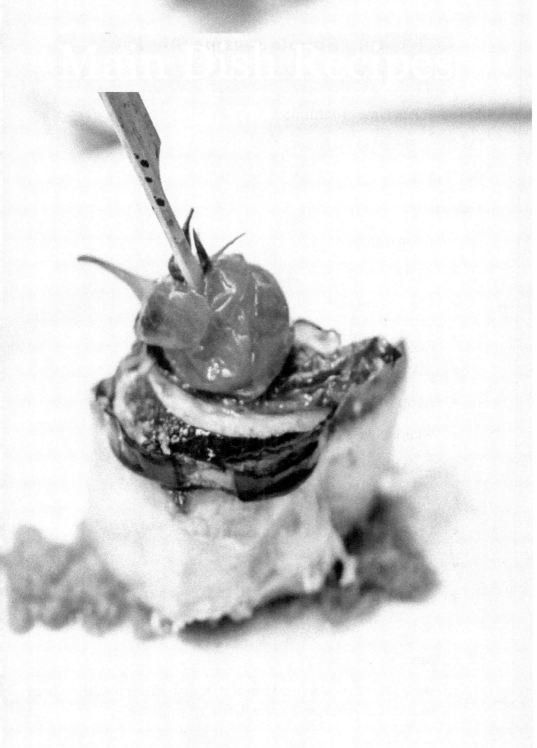

10. Simple Sesame Stir-Fry

Preparation Time: 10 minutes

Cooking Time: 20 minutes

Serving: 4

Ingredient:

- 1 cup quinoa
- 2 cups water
- 1 head broccoli
- 2 teaspoons olive oil
- 1 cup snow peas
- 1 cup peas
- 2 cups Swiss chard
- 2 scallions
- 2 tablespoons water
- 1 teaspoon toasted sesame oil
- 1 tablespoon tamari
- 2 tablespoons sesame seeds

Directions:

1. Boil quinoa, water, and sea salt in a medium pot, then turn to low and simmer, covered, for 20 minutes.

2. Cut broccoli into bite-size florets, cutting and pulling apart from the stem. Also chop the stem into bite-size pieces.

3. Heat a large skillet to high, and sauté the broccoli in the untoasted sesame oil, with a dash of salt to help it soften. Put the snow peas next, continuing to stir. Add the edamame until they thaw. Add the Swiss chard and scallions at the same time, tossing for only a minute to wilt. Then add 2 tablespoons of water to the hot skillet so that it sizzles and finishes the vegetables with a quick steam.

4. Dress with the toasted sesame oil and tamari, and toss one last time. Remove from the heat immediately.

5. Serve a scoop of cooked quinoa, topped with stir-fry and sprinkled with some sesame seeds.

Nutrition:

334 Calories

9g Fiber

17g Protein

11. Sun-dried Tomato and Pesto Quinoa

Preparation Time: 10 minutes

Cooking Time: 15 minutes

Serving: 1

Ingredients:

- 1 teaspoon olive oil
- 1 cup d onion
- 1 garlic clove
- 1 cup zucchini
- 1 tomato
- 2 tablespoons sun-dried tomatoes
- 3 tablespoons Basil Pesto
- 1 cup spinach
- 2 cups cooked quinoa

Direction:

1. Cook oil in a big skillet on medium-high, then sauté the onion, about 5 minutes. Stir in garlic when the onion has softened, then add the zucchini and salt.

2. Once the zucchini is somewhat soft, about 5 minutes, turn off the heat and add the fresh and sun-dried tomatoes. Mix

to combine, then toss in the pesto. Toss the vegetables to coat them.

3. Layer the spinach, then quinoa, then the zucchini mixture on a plate, topped with a bit of Cheesy Sprinkle (if using).

Nutrition:

535 Calories

14g Fiber

20g Protei

12. Olive and White Bean Pasta

Preparation Time: 10 minutes

Cooking Time: 20 minutes

Serving: 1

Ingredient:

- ½ cup whole-grain pasta
- 1 teaspoon olive oil
- ¼ cup red bell pepper
- ¼ cup zucchini
- ½ cup cannellini beans
- ½ cup spinach
- 1 tablespoon balsamic vinegar
- 3 black olives
- 1 tablespoon nutritional yeast

Direction:

1. Boil water, then add the pasta with the salt to cook until just tender (per the package directions).

2. In a big skillet, cook oil and lightly sauté the bell pepper and zucchini, 7 to 8 minutes. Add the beans to warm for 2 minutes, then add the spinach last, just until it wilts. Drizzle with the vinegar at the end.

3. Serve the pasta topped or tossed with the bean mixture, and sprinkled with the olives and nutritional yeast.

Nutrition:

387 Calories

19g Fiber

18g Protein

13. BBQ Fruit Sliders

Preparation Time: 13 minutes

Cooking Time: 12 minutes

Serving: 5

Ingredient:

- 2 (20-ounce) cans young green jackfruit
- ½ cup BBQ Sauce
- 1 teaspoon garlic powder
- 1 teaspoon onion powder
- 6 whole-wheat slider buns
- Asian-Style Slaw with Maple-Ginger Dressing, for topping

Direction:

1. Smash the jackfruit until it has a shredded consistency.

2. Heat a medium stockpot over medium-low heat. Put the shredded jackfruit, BBQ sauce, garlic powder, and onion powder in the pot, and stir. Cook for 10 minutes, covered, stirring once after about 5 minutes. If the jackfruit begins sticking to the bottom of the pot, add in a few tablespoons of vegetable broth or water.

3. Uncover and cook for 5 minutes, stirring every few minutes.

4. Serve on whole-wheat slider buns with your favorite toppings.

Nutrition:

188 Calories

36g Carbohydrates

7g Protein

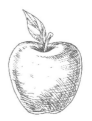

14. Hawaiian Luau Burgers

Preparation Time: 15 minutes

Cooking Time: 10 minutes

Serving: 8

Ingredients:

- 3 cups cooked black beans
- 2 cups cooked brown rice
- 1 cup quick-cooking oats
- ¼ cup BBQ Sauce
- ¼ cup pineapple juice
- 1 teaspoon garlic powder
- 1 teaspoon onion powder
- 1 pineapple
- 8 whole-wheat buns

Direction:

1. Preheat the grill to medium-high heat.
2. Mash the black beans.
3. Incorporate rice, oats, BBQ sauce, the pineapple juice, garlic powder, and onion powder to form into patties.
4. Spoon out ½ cup of bean mixture, and form it into a patty. Repeat.

5. Grill patties for 4 minutes on 1 side, flipping once the burgers easily release from the grill surface.

6. After grilling, cook pineapple rings 1 to 2 minutes on each side.

7. Stack one patty and one pineapple ring with a spoonful of the BBQ sauce and serve.

Nutrition:

371 Calories

71g Carbohydrates

15g Protein

15. Falafel Burgers

Preparation Time: 15 minutes

Cooking Time: 30 minutes

Serving: 8

Ingredient:

- 3 cups chickpeas
- 2 cups brown rice
- ¼ cup vegetable broth
- ¼ cup chopped fresh parsley
- 1 tablespoon lemon juice
- 2 teaspoons garlic powder
- 2 teaspoons onion powder
- 1½ teaspoons ground cumin
- 1 teaspoon ground coriander
- ¼ teaspoon black pepper
- whole-wheat buns

Direction:

1. Preheat the oven to 425°F. Line a baking sheet with parchment paper.

2. Blend chickpeas, rice, broth, parsley, lemon juice, garlic powder, onion powder, cumin, coriander, and pepper on low for 40 seconds.

3. Scoop out ½ cup of the chickpea mixture, and form it into a patty. Place the patty on the baking sheet. Repeat.

4. Bake for 15 minutes. Flip the patties, cook for 15 minutes more, and serve buns with your preferred toppings.

Nutrition:

230 Calories

44g Carbohydrates

10g Protein

16. Crispy Rice-and-Bean Tostadas

Preparation Time: 10 minutes

Cooking Time: 10 minutes

Serving: 2

Ingredient:

- 4 corn tortillas
- 1 cup Fat-Free Refried Beans
- 1 cup brown rice
- 1 cup black beans
- 1 lime

Direction:

1. Preheat the oven to 400°F. Line a baking sheet with parchment paper.
2. Bake tortillas for 7 minutes.
3. Evenly spread ¼ cup of refried beans onto each crispy tortilla, then add ¼ cup each of rice and black beans.
4. Squeeze lime juice over each tostada right before serving.

Nutrition:

422 Calories

19g Fiber

19g Protein

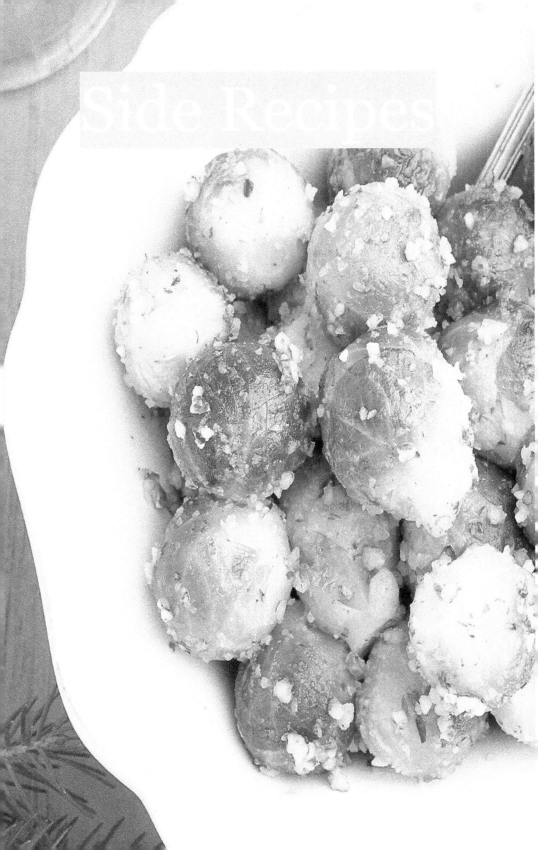

17. Moroccan Chickpea Stew

Preparation Time: 15 minutes

Cooking Time: 6 hours

Serving: 4

Ingredients:

- 1 small butternut squash
- 3 cups Very Easy Vegetable Broth
- 1 medium yellow onion
- 1 bell pepper
- 1 (15-ounce) can chickpeas
- 1 (14.5-ounce) can tomato sauce
- ¾ cup brown lentils
- 1½ teaspoons garlic
- 1½ teaspoons ground ginger
- 1½ teaspoons ground turmeric
- 1½ teaspoons ground cumin
- 1 teaspoon ground cinnamon
- ¾ teaspoon smoked paprika
- ½ teaspoon salt
- 1 (8-ounce) package fresh udon noodles

Direction

1. Incorporate butternut squash, vegetable broth, onion, bell pepper, chickpeas, tomato sauce, brown lentils, garlic, ginger, turmeric, cumin, cinnamon, smoked paprika, and salt in a slow cooker. Mix well.

2. Cover and cook 6 hours on low. Stir in noodles. Season and serve.

Nutrition:

427 Calories

26g Protein

24g Fiber

18. Tex-Mex Taco Filling

Preparation Time: 15 minutes

Cooking Time: 7 hours

Serving: 6

Ingredient:

- 2 cups Very Easy Vegetable Broth
- 1 cup green lentils
- ½ cup uncooked quinoa
- ¼ cup yellow onion
- 1½ teaspoons garlic
- 2 teaspoons ground cumin
- 1 teaspoon chili powder
- ½ teaspoon smoked paprika

Direction:

1. Blend vegetable broth, lentils, quinoa, onion, garlic, cumin, chili powder, and smoked paprika in a slow cooker.

2. Cook in low for 7 hours. Season. Serve with your choice of toppings.

Nutrition: 14g Protein

283 Calories   17g Fiber

19. Cauliflower Bolognese

Preparation Time: 15 minutes

Cooking Time: 9 hours

Serving: 4

Ingredient:

- ½ head cauliflower
- 1 (10-ounce) container button mushrooms
- 1 small yellow onion
- 2 medium carrots
- 2 cups eggplant chunks
- 2½ teaspoons garlic
- 2 (28-ounce) cans tomatoes
- 2 tablespoons tomato paste
- 2 tablespoons cane sugar
- 2 tablespoons balsamic vinegar
- 2 tablespoons nutritional yeast
- 1½ tablespoons dried oregano
- 1½ tablespoons dried basil
- 1½ teaspoons fresh rosemary leaves

Direction

1. In a food processor, blend cauliflower, mushrooms, onion, carrots, eggplant, and garlic. Transfer to a slow cooker.

2. Add the crushed tomatoes, tomato paste, cane sugar, balsamic vinegar, nutritional yeast, oregano, basil, and rosemary to the slow cooker; mix well.

3. Cover and cook in low for 9 hours. Season and serve.

Nutrition:

281 Calories

17g Protein

10g Fiber

20. Veggie Spring Rolls

Preparation Time: 15 minutes

Cooking Time: 5 minutes

Serving: 4

Ingredients:

- 3 cups water
- 1 (8-ounce) package thin rice noodles
- 1 (8-ounce) jar peanut sauce
- 1 large cucumber
- 2 small red bell peppers
- 8 rice wrappers

Direction:

1. Boil water. Place the rice noodles and pour the hot water. Let sit for 3 minutes. Drain, and pour the peanut sauce over the noodles. Toss; set aside.

2. Leaving the peel on the cucumber, cut it in half and then julienne each half to create 16 (¼-inch-wide) sticks.

3. Slice circle around the top of each red pepper. Cut off stem and seeds. Cut each into four parts, then slice into 16 strips total.

4. Dip 1 rice wrapper in warm water for 5 seconds. Place the moist rice wrapper on a work surface and let sit for 30 seconds. Add one eighth of the noodles and sauce, 2

cucumber sticks, and 2 pepper strips. Lift one side of the rice wrapper and fold over the filling, tucking it under the filling. Crease in the sides and continue rolling until you come to the end of the wrapper. Repeat process.

Nutrition:

551 Calories

6g Fiber

13g Protein

21. Smoky Coleslaw

Preparation Time: 10 minutes

Cooking Time: 0 minute

Serving: 4

Ingredients:

- 1-pound cabbage
- ½ cup plain vegan yogurt
- ¼ cup unseasoned rice vinegar
- 1 tablespoon sugar
- ½ teaspoon smoked paprika

Direction:

1. Puree yogurt, vinegar, sugar, paprika, salt, and pepper.
2. Drizzle dressing over the cabbage and mix Cover and chill for an hour.

Nutrition:

62 Calories

3g Fiber

2g Protein

22. Baked Ratatouille

Preparation Time: 10 minutes

Cooking Time: 36 minutes

Servings 4

Ingredients:

- 1 large zucchini
- 1 small eggplant
- 2 teaspoons olive oil
- 1 small red onion
- 1 (24-ounce) jar marinara sauce
- ½ cup basil leaves

Direction:

1. Preheat the oven to 400°F.

2. Slice the zucchini and eggplant (peel on) into ¼-inch rounds. Set aside.

3. Warm up olive oil over medium-high heat. Sauté onion. Cook marinara sauce for 3 minutes.

4. Reserve ¾ cup of the sauce and transfer the rest of it to an 8-inch square baking pan with 2-inch sides. Arrange the basil over the sauce. Place the zucchini and eggplant rounds over the basil and sauce. Dash rest 1 teaspoon olive oil over the vegetables and season Pour the reserved ¾ cup sauce over everything.

5. Seal with foil and bake it for 20 minutes. Remove then bake for 10 minutes.

Nutrition:

123 Calories

8g Fiber

5g Protein

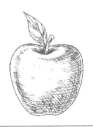

23. Pea Nutty Carrot Noodles

Preparation Time: 5 minutes

Cooking Time: 2 minutes

Serving: 4

Ingredient:

- 1 teaspoon olive oil
- 3 large carrots
- 1 small lime
- ½ teaspoon salt
- ½ cup peanuts
- ½ cup chopped scallions

Direction:

1. Over medium-high heat, heat the olive oil. Cook carrots, cover for 2 minutes. Remove from the heat, mix lime juice and salt, and toss.

2. To serve, top each with 2 tablespoons peanuts and 2 tablespoons scallions.

Nutrition: 3g Fiber

142 Calories   5g Protein

Vegetable

Recipes

24. Raw Nut Cheese

Preparation Time: 10 minutes + 12 hours soak time

Cooking Time: 0 min.

Servings: 3

Ingredients:

- 3 2/3 cups raw cashews
- 1 teaspoon of probiotic powder
- 2 tablespoons onion powder
- 1 tablespoon garlic powder
- 4-5 tablespoons nutritional yeast

Direction:

1. Drain the water from the overnight soaked cashews. Put them in a blender with the probiotic powder, blending until smooth.

2. Wrap mixture with plastic wrap or beeswax wrap, being careful to leave a couple tiny spaces open for air to get in. Leave the bowl at room temperature for 8-12 hours, or until the cheese has risen in size.

3. Sprinkle with the onion powder, garlic powder, nutritional yeast, salt, and pepper.

Nutrition: 36g Protein

890 Calories   65g Fat

25. Italian Tomatoes

Preparation Time: 7 minutes

Cooking Time: 3 minutes

Servings: 3

Ingredients:

- 2 large, ripe tomatoes
- 1 teaspoon red wine vinegar
- 4 thin slices of sourdough bread
- ½ garlic clove
- 1 teaspoon extra virgin olive oil

Directions:

1. Begin toasting the bread on a hot griddle, or slightly warm the paleo bread you've made from the recipe above it if you're following a raw diet.
2. Wash and chop the tomatoes.
3. Mix the tomatoes with the vinegar, salt and pepper.
4. Press the garlic, crushing it into a fine pulp. Spread very thinly on the toast. Top the toast with the tomatoes and add a bit of olive oil on top of each. Consume immediately.

Nutrition: 6.4g Protein

212 Calories   2.8g Fat

26. Gluten-Free, Raw Bread with Caraway Onion

Preparation Time: 15 minutes

Cooking Time: 0 minute

Serving: 4

Ingredients:

- 4 ½ ounces sunflower seeds

- 3 ounces walnuts

- 3 celery stalks

- 2 ounces raisins

- 1 red onion

- 2 teaspoons caraway seeds

- 2 tablespoons ground coriander

- 2 pinches Himalayan salt

- 3 ounces ground flaxseeds

- 4 ounces extra virgin olive oil

- 4 tablespoons lemon juice

Direction:

1. Submerge seeds and nuts overnight or for 4-6 hours. Drain the water. Dice the onion, celery and chop the seeds. Add

all into a blender or food processor and mix very well for 2-5 minutes or until well blended. Add the rest of the ingredients.

2. Pat out flat on a baking tray lined with wax paper, or put into a dehydrator. Bake at 115°F for 6 hours.

Nutrition:

212 Calories

6.4g Protein

2.8g Fat

27. Chipotle, Pinto, and Green Bean

Preparation Time: 5 minutes

Cooking Time: 10 minutes

Serving: 2

Ingredient:

- 2 tablespoons extra-virgin olive oil
- 1½ cups fresh or frozen corn
- 1 cup green beans, chopped
- 2 green onions
- ½ tablespoon garlic
- 1 medium tomato
- 1 teaspoon chili powder
- ½ teaspoon chipotle powder
- ½ teaspoon ground cumin
- 1 (14-ounce) can pinto beans
- 1 teaspoon sea salt

Direction

1. Cook olive oil in a huge skillet over medium heat. Add the corn, green beans, green onions, and garlic and stir for 5 minutes.

2. Add the tomato, chili powder, chipotle powder, and cumin and stir for 3 minutes, until the tomato starts to soften. In a bowl, mash some of the pinto beans with a fork. Add all of the beans to the skillet and stir for 2 minutes

3. Pull away from the heat and stir in the salt. Serve hot or warm.

Nutrition:

391 Calories

15g Fiber

15g Protein

28. Mixed Vegetable Medley

Preparation Time: 5 minutes

Cooking Time: 20 minutes

Serving: 2

Ingredient:

- 1 stick (½ cup) unsalted butter
- 1 large potato
- 1 onion
- ½ tablespoon garlic
- 1 cup green beans
- 2 ears fresh sweet corn
- 1 red bell pepper
- 2 cups white mushrooms

Direction:

1. Warm up half of the butter in a large nonstick skillet over medium-high heat. When the butter is frothy, add the potato and cook, stirring frequently, for 15 minutes.

2. Mix in rest of butter, turn down the heat to medium, and add the onion, garlic, green beans, and corn. Cook, stirring frequently, for 5 minutes.

3. Add the red bell pepper and mushrooms. Stir for another 5 minutes. Add more butter, if necessary.

4. Pull out from heat and season. Serve hot.

Nutrition:

688 Calories

11g Fiber

11g Protein

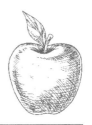

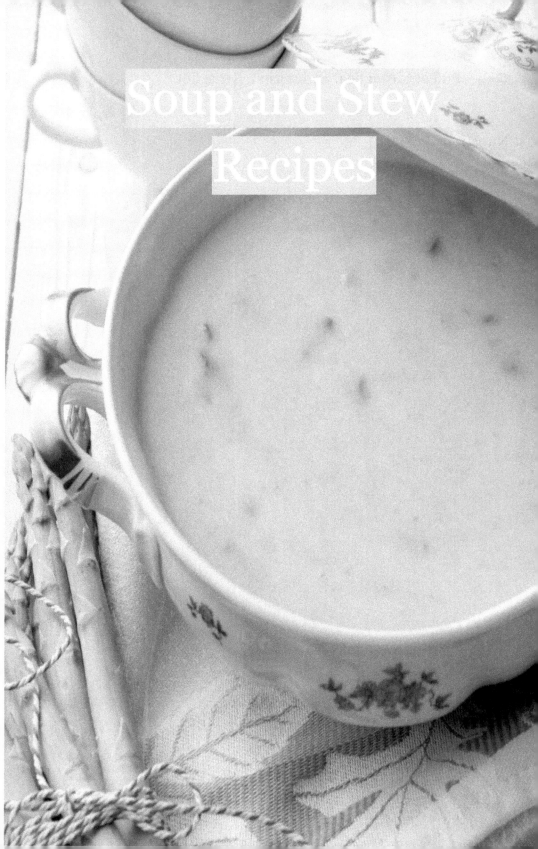

Soup and Stew

Recipes

29. African Pineapple Peanut Stew

Preparation Time: 10 minutes

Cooking Time: 20 minutes

Servings: 4

Ingredients:

- 4 cups kale
- 1 cup onion
- ½ cup peanut butter
- 1 tbsp. hot pepper sauce
- 2 minced garlic cloves
- ½ cup chopped cilantro
- 2 cups pineapple
- 1 tbsp. vegetable oil

Directions:

1. In a saucepan sauté the garlic and onions in the oil until the onions are lightly browned, approximately 10 minutes, stirring often.

2. Wash the kale, till the time the onions are sauté.

3. Get rid of the stems. Mound the leaves on a cutting surface & slice crosswise into slices (preferably 1" thick).

4. Now put the pineapple and juice to the onions & bring to a simmer. Stir the kale in, cover and simmer until just tender, stirring frequently, approximately 5 minutes.

5. Mix in the hot pepper sauce, peanut butter & simmer for more 5 minutes.

6. Add salt according to your taste.

Nutrition:

193 Calories

10g Protein

7g Fiber

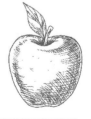

30. Cabbage & Beet Stew

Preparation Time: 20 minutes

Cooking Time: 10 minutes

Servings: 4

Ingredients:

- 2 Tablespoons Olive Oil
- 3 Cups Vegetable Broth
- 2 Tablespoons Lemon Juice, Fresh
- ½ Teaspoon Garlic Powder
- ½ Cup Carrots
- 2 Cups Cabbage
- 1 Cup Beets
- Dill for Garnish
- ½ Teaspoon Onion Powder

Directions:

1. Heat oil in a pot, and then sauté your vegetables.
2. Pour your broth in, mixing in your seasoning. Simmer then tops with dill.

Nutrition: 8g Protein

173 Calories   6g Fiber

31.   Basil Tomato Soup

Preparation Time: 10 minutes

Cooking Time: 10 minutes

Servings: 6

Ingredients:

- 28 oz. can tomato
- ¼ cup basil pesto
- ¼ tsp. dried basil leaves
- 1 tsp. apple cider vinegar
- 2 tbsp. erythritol
- ¼ tsp. garlic powder
- ½ tsp. onion powder
- 2 cups water
- 1 ½ tsp. kosher salt

Directions:

1. Add tomatoes, garlic powder, onion powder, water, and salt in a saucepan.

2. Bring to boil over medium heat. Reduce heat and simmer for 2 minutes.

3. Pull out saucepan from heat and mash soup using a blender until smooth.

4. Stir well pesto, dried basil, vinegar, and erythritol.

Nutrition:

163 Calories

12g Protein

32. 5gg Fiber

33. Hearty Chickpea Soup

Preparation Time: 10 minutes

Cooking Time: 10 minutes

Serving: 7

Ingredient:

- 2 carrots
- 4 celery stalks
- 6 cups Economical Vegetable Broth
- 8 cups water
- 8 ounces spaghetti or thin brown rice noodles
- 1½ cups cooked chickpeas
- 1 teaspoon dried herbs
- ¼ to ½ teaspoon salt

Direction:

1. In a huge soup pot, mix carrots, celery, vegetable broth, and water. Bring to a boil over medium heat, then add the spaghetti, chickpeas, dried herbs, ¼ teaspoon salt (or ½ teaspoon if your broth is unsalted), and a few grinds of pepper. Cook for 9 minutes.

Nutrition: 8g Protein

173 Calories   6g Fiber

34. Cream of Tomato Soup

Preparation Time: 5 minutes

Cooking Time: 5 minutes

Serving: 2

Ingredient:

- 1 (28-ounce) can tomatoes

- 2 teaspoons dried herbs

- 3 teaspoons onion powder

- 1 cup unsweetened nondairy milk

Direction:

1. Fill tomatoes and their juices into a large pot and bring them to near-boiling over medium heat. Add the dried herbs, onion powder (if using), milk, salt, and pepper to taste. Stir to combine.

2. Mix tomatoes, use a hand blender to purée the soup.

Nutrition

90 Calories

4g Protein

4g Fiber

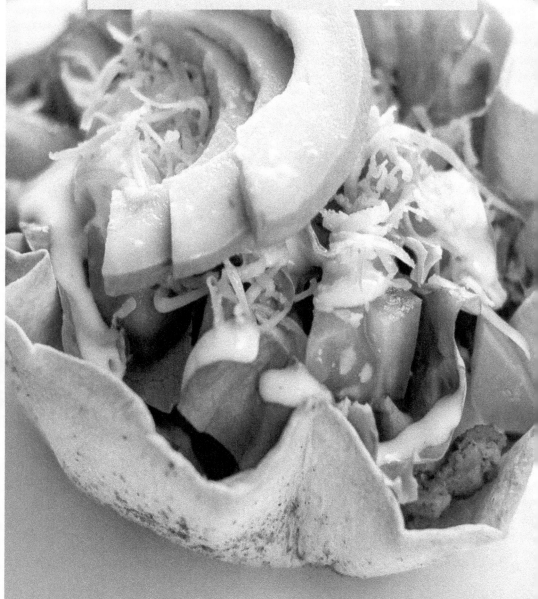

Salad Recipes

35. Quinoa Pilaf

Preparation Time: 10 minutes

Cooking Time: 15 minutes

Serving: 4

Ingredients:

- 1 cup quinoa

- 2 cups vegetable stock

- ¼ cup pine nuts

- 2 tablespoons olive oil

- ½ onion

- 1/3 cup parsley

Direction:

1. In a pot, boil quinoa and vegetable stock over medium-high heat, stirring occasionally. Reduce to a simmer. Cover and cook for 15 minutes.

2. Preheat sauté pan over medium-high heat. Toast pine nuts to the dry hot pan for 3 minutes. Keep aside.

3. Fill olive oil to the same pan and heat until it shimmers. Cook onion for 5 minutes.

4. When the quinoa is soft and all the liquid is absorbed, remove it from the heat and fluff it with a fork. Stir in the pine nuts, onion, and parsley. Season with salt and -pepper. Serve hot.

Nutrition:

188 Calories

10g Protein

3g Fiber

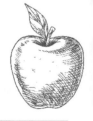

36. Lemon and Thyme Couscous

Preparation Time: 5 minutes

Cooking Time: 10 minutes

Serving: 6

Ingredients:

- 2¾ cups vegetable stock
- Juice and zest of 1 lemon
- 2 tablespoons thyme
- 1½ cups couscous
- ¼ cup parsley

Direction:

1. In a medium pot, boil together vegetable stock, lemon juice, and thyme. Stir in the couscous, cover, and remove from the heat. Keep aside for 5 minutes. Fluff with a fork.

2. Stir in the lemon zest and parsley. Season with salt and pepper. Serve hot.

Nutrition:

288 Calories

5g Protein

4g Fiber

37. Spicy Picnic Beans

Preparation Time: 15 minutes

Cooking Time: 15 minutes

Serving: 6

Ingredients:

- 1 jalapeño
- 1 red bell pepper
- 1 green bell pepper
- 1 onion
- 5 garlic cloves
- Two 15-ounce cans pinto beans
- One 15-ounce can kidney beans
- One 15-ounce can chickpeas
- One 18-ounce bottle barbecue sauce
- ½ teaspoon chipotle powder

Direction:

1. In food processor, blend jalapeño, bell peppers, onion, and garlic for ten 1-second pulses, stopping halfway through to scrape down the sides.

2. In a large pot, combine the processed mixture with the beans, barbecue sauce, and chipotle powder. Simmer over medium-high heat, stirring frequently to blend the flavors, about 15 minutes.

3. Season with salt and pepper. Serve hot.

Nutrition:

178 Calories

11g Protein

5g Fiber

38. Chickpeas with Lemon and Spinach

Preparation Time: 8 minutes

Cooking Time: 12 minutes

Serving: 3

Ingredients:

- 3 tablespoons olive oil
- One 15-ounce can chickpeas
- 10 ounces baby spinach
- ½ teaspoon sea salt
- Juice and zest of 1 lemon

Direction:

1. In a huge sauté pan, preheat olive oil over medium-high heat until it shimmers. Cook chickpeas for 5 minutes.

2. Cook spinach for 5 minutes. Add the salt, lemon juice, lemon zest, and pepper and stir to combine. Serve immediately.

Nutrition: 11g Protein

208 Calories   7g Fiber

39. Spicy Chickpeas

Preparation Time: 10 minutes

Cooking Time: 35 minutes

Servings: 6

Ingredients:

- ¼ cup olive oil
- ½ tsp. cayenne pepper
- 2 (15 oz.) chickpeas
- ¾ tsp. paprika
- 1 tsp. sea salt
- ½ tsp. chili powder
- ½ tsp. onion powder
- ½ tsp. cumin
- ¾ tsp. garlic powder

Directions:

1. Ready oven to 425 degrees F. Strain chickpeas and let them dry in a towel-lined dish for 10 to 15 minutes. Transfer the chickpeas onto a lined baking sheet and spread them out in a single layer.

2. Pour olive oil over the chickpeas and sprinkle with salt. Bake them in the oven for 23 to 25 minutes or until they are golden brown, stirring frequently.

3. Once baked, stir in the remaining spices and toss well. Next, season and taste, adding more salt and pepper as needed. Serve and enjoy.

Nutrition:

224 Calories

13g Protein

10g Fat

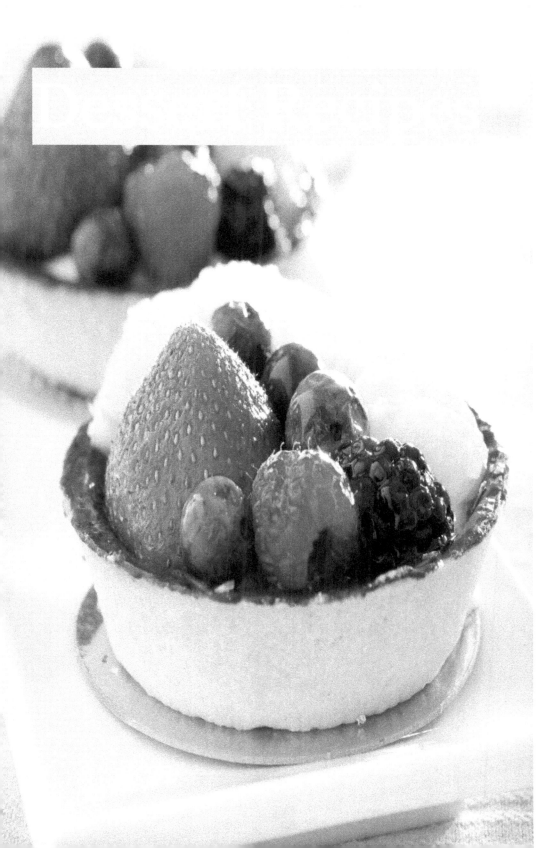

40. Chocolate Macaroons

Preparation Time: 10 minutes

Cooking Time: 15 minutes

Servings: 8

Ingredients

- 1 cup unsweetened coconut
- 2 tablespoons cocoa powder
- 2/3 Cup coconut milk
- ¼ Cup agave

Directions:

1. Preheat the oven to 350°f. Line a baking sheet with parchment paper. In a medium saucepan, cook all the Ingredients over -medium-high heat until a firm dough is formed. Scoop the dough into balls and place on the baking sheet.

2. Bake for 15 minutes, remove from the oven, and let cool on the baking sheet.

3. Serve cooled macaroons or store in a tightly sealed container for up to

Nutrition   5g protein

119 calories   4g fiber

41. Chocolate Pudding

Preparation Time: 7 minutes

Cooking Time: 0 minute

Servings: 2

Ingredients

- 1 banana
- 2 to 4 tablespoons nondairy milk
- 2 tablespoons unsweetened cocoa powder
- 2 tablespoons sugar
- ½ Ripe avocado

Directions:

1. In a small blender, combine the banana, milk, cocoa powder, sugar (if using), and avocado (if using). Purée until smooth.

Nutrition

244 calories

4g protein

8g fiber

42.   Lime and Watermelon

Preparation Time: 17 minutes

Cooking Time: 0 minute

Servings: 5

Ingredients

- 8 cups seedless -watermelon chunks
- Juice of 2 limes
- ½ Cup sugar
- Strips of lime zest, for garnish

Directions:

1. In a blender or food processor, combine the watermelon, lime juice, and sugar and process until smooth. You may have to do this in two batches. After processing, stir well to combine both batches.

2. Pour the mixture into a 9-by-13-inch glass dish. Freeze for 2 to 3 hours. Remove from the freezer and use a fork to scrape the top layer of ice. Leave the shaved ice on top and return to the freezer.

3. In another hour, remove from the freezer and repeat. Do this a few more times until all the ice is scraped up. Serve frozen, garnished with strips of lime zest.

Nutrition   8g protein

124 calories   3g fibeR

43. Coconut-Banana Pudding

Preparation Time: 4 minutes

Cooking Time: 5 minutes

Servings: 4

Ingredients

- 3 bananas
- 1 (13.5-ounce) can full-fat coconut milk
- ¼ Cup organic cane sugar
- 1 tablespoon cornstarch
- 1 teaspoon vanilla extract
- 2 pinches salt
- 6 drops natural yellow food coloring

Directions:

1. Combine 1 banana, the coconut milk, sugar, cornstarch, vanilla, and salt in a blender. Blend until smooth and creamy.

2. Transfer to a saucepot and bring to a boil over medium-high heat. Immediately reduce to a simmer and whisk for 3 minutes.

3. Transfer the mixture to a container and allow to cool for 1 hour. Cover and refrigerate overnight to set. When you're ready to serve, slice the remaining 2 bananas and

build individual servings as follows: pudding, banana slices, pudding, and so on until a single-serving dish is filled to the desired level. Sprinkle with ground cinnamon.

Nutrition

109 calories

8g protein

4g fiber

44. Beets Bars with Dry Fruits

Preparation Time: 10 minutes

Cooking Time: 40 minutes

Serving: 4

Ingredients

- 1 Tbsp. flax seed
- 3 Tbsp. water
- 5 oz. whole wheat flour
- 8 ounces beetroot
- 3 Tbsp. dates
- 3 Tbsp. figs
- 4 Tbsp. honey
- 4 Tbsp. olive oil
- 1 tsp. baking powder
- 1 tsp. baking soda
- 1 tsp. pure vanilla extract
- 1/4 tsp. salt

Direction:

1. Preheat oven to 300F.

2. Soak the flaxseed with water for 10 minutes.

3. Grease a baking sheet with olive oil; set aside.

4. Place the wheat flour along with all remaining ingredients into a food processor.

5. Process until all ingredients are combined well.

6. Place the mixture into the prepared baking sheet and bake for 35 to 40 minutes.

7. Remove the baking sheet from the oven, and let it cool completely.

8. Cut into squares and serve.

9. Store into a container and refrigerate up to 4 days.

Nutrition

247 Calories

1.8g Fiber

3.1g Protein

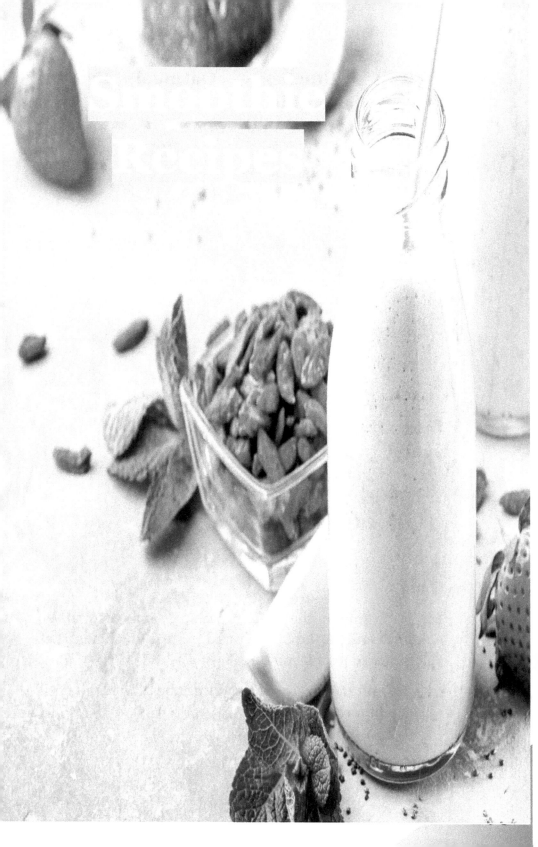

45. Blueberry Oatmeal Protein Smoothie

Preparation Time: 15 minutes

Cooking Time: 0 minute

Serving: 3

Ingredients:

- ½ cup water
- ½ cup rolled oats
- 1 cup almond milk
- 1 cup blueberries
- 4 ice cubes
- 1 scoop vanilla protein powder
- 2 tablespoons chia seed
- 1 tablespoon almond butter

Directions:

1.   Combine the water, oatmeal and coconut or almond milk in the blender and pulse a few times. Let sit for three to four minutes.

2.   Add the blueberries and ice cubes and blend until just combined.

3.   Add the protein powder, ground chia seeds and almond butter. Blend until everything is smooth and thick. Add more ice if needed to balance the consistency.

Nutrition

195 Calories

6g Fiber

8g Protein

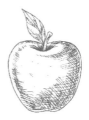

46. Carrot Orange Smoothie

Preparation Time: 11 minutes

Cooking Time: 0 minute

Serving: 2

Ingredients:

- 2 tablespoons flax seeds
- ½ cup unsweetened coconut milk
- 2 oranges, peeled, sections separated and frozen
- 1-inch ginger, peeled and grated
- 2 large carrots, peeled then cut into small chunks

Directions:

1. Grind the chia seeds with a coffee grinder and place them in the blender.

2. Pour in the coconut milk and frozen orange segments; pulse to mix until chunky.

3. Add the ginger and carrots, blending until smooth and creamy.

Nutrition   11g Protein

210 Calories

9g Fiber

47. Chocolate-Strawberry Heaven

Preparation Time: 15 minutes

Cooking Time: 0 minute

Serving: 2

Ingredients:

- 1 tablespoon chia seeds, ground

- 1 cup almond milk

- 1 scoop chocolate protein powder

- 2 tablespoons raw almonds

- 1 cup frozen, sliced strawberries

Directions:

1. Grind the chia seeds and place them in a blender with the almond milk.

2. Add the chocolate protein powder and almonds and pulse mix everything together.

3. Add the strawberries and blend until smooth and rich and thick.

Nutrition

209 Calories

8g Fiber

9g Protein

48. Cherry Limeade Smoothie

Preparation Time: 10 minutes

Cooking Time: 0 minute

Serving: 2

Ingredients:

- 1 heaping cup of frozen pitted cherries
- 1 ripe peach, peeled and sliced
- 1 tablespoon ground chia seeds
- 1 cup almond milk
- 1 to 2 limes, juiced
- 1 handful of ice

Directions:

1.   Add the cherries and peach slices to the blender and pulse.

2.   Add the ground chia seeds and pulse.

3.   Pour in the almond milk, lime juice and ice; blend until smooth and thick. Add ice if more thickness is needed.

Nutrition   10g Fiber

211 Calories

49. Mint Protein Smoothie

Preparation Time: 10 minutes

Cooking Time: 0 minute

Serving: 2

Ingredients:

- 1 tablespoon chia seeds, ground
- 1 tablespoon hemp seeds, ground
- 1 tablespoon flax seed, ground
- ½ cup mango pieces, frozen
- 1 large orange, peeled and sectioned
- 1 banana, peeled, chopped in pieces and frozen
- 1 scoop vanilla protein powder
- ¾ cup unsweetened coconut milk
- 6 fresh mint leaves

Directions:

1.   Grind the chia, hemp and flax seed and place them in a blender.

2.   Add the frozen mango, the orange sections and the frozen banana pieces to the blender and pulse a few times.

3.   Add the protein powder and coconut milk; pulse again to combine.

4. Add the mint leaves and blend until smooth. If the smoothie is too runny, add a few ice cubes and blend again until thick and smooth.

Nutrition

204 Calories

4g Fiber

9g Protein

30-Day Meal Plan

DAY	BREAKFAST	MAIN DISH	SIDE	DESSERT
1	chocolate zoats	simple sesame stir-fry	moroccan chickpea stew	chocolate pudding
2	greens on toast with tofu ricotta	sun-dried tomato and pesto quinoa	tex-mex taco filling	chocolate macaroons
3	chocolate zoats	bbq fruit sliders	veggie spring rolls	coconut-banana pudding
4	cashew cheese spread	simple sesame stir-fry	cauliflower bolognese	lime and watermelon
5	staple smoothie	falafel burgers	baked ratatouille	chocolate pudding
6	cashew cheese spread	bbq fruit sliders	baked ratatouille	beets bars with dry fruits
7	greens on toast with tofu ricotta	olive and white bean pasta	cauliflower bolognese	chocolate macaroons

8	chocolate zoats	sun-dried tomato and pesto quinoa	moroccan chickpea stew	chocolate pudding
9	staple smoothie	olive and white bean pasta	tex-mex taco filling	chocolate macaroons
10	fruit and nut oatmeal	falafel burgers	moroccan chickpea stew	lime and watermelon
11	chocolate zoats	hawaiian luau burgers	cauliflower bolognese	beets bars with dry fruits
12	fruit and nut oatmeal	bbq fruit sliders	tex-mex taco filling	beets bars with dry fruits
13	greens on toast with tofu ricotta	simple sesame stir-fry	tex-mex taco filling	coconut-banana pudding
14	chocolate zoats	simple sesame stir-fry	moroccan chickpea stew	coconut-banana pudding
15	cashew cheese spread	falafel burgers	veggie spring rolls	chocolate pudding

16	greens on toast with tofu ricotta	sun-dried tomato and pesto quinoa	veggie spring rolls	chocolate macaroons
17	chocolate zoats	falafel burgers	moroccan chickpea stew	beets bars with dry fruits
18	cashew cheese spread	bbq fruit sliders	baked ratatouille	coconut-banana pudding
19	staple smoothie	falafel burgers	tex-mex taco filling	lime and watermelon
20	fruit and nut oatmeal	simple sesame stir-fry	veggie spring rolls	chocolate pudding
21	Chocolate zoats	Olive and white bean pasta	Cauliflower bolognese	Coconut-banana pudding
22	Cashew cheese spread	Sun-dried tomato and pesto quinoa	Moroccan chickpea stew	Chocolate macaroons

23	Greens on toast with tofu ricotta	Bbq fruit sliders	Tex-mex taco filling	Lime and watermelon
24	chocolate zoats	simple sesame stir-fry	moroccan chickpea stew	chocolate pudding
25	staple smoothie	sun-dried tomato and pesto quinoa	veggie spring rolls	lime and watermelon
26	cashew cheese spread	hawaiian luau burgers	veggie spring rolls	chocolate macaroons
27	staple smoothie	olive and white bean pasta	cauliflower bolognese	chocolate macaroons
28	chocolate zoats	hawaiian luau burgers	tex-mex taco filling	lime and watermelon
29	fruit and nut oatmeal	sun-dried tomato	moroccan chickpea stew	chocolate macaroons
30	greens on toast with tofu ricotta	Simple Sesame Stir-Fry	Veggie Spring Rolls	Coconut-Banana Pudding

Conclusion

As an athlete, it may sound like the vegan diet may not provide you the right nutrition. Rest assured; you can very well debunk that myth.

Over the course of the book, I've given you a bunch of tasty and easy to make recipes that will surely provide you fair share of carbohydrates and protein. Keep in mind that being meat-free athlete isn't simple, this is barely a reason to quit!

One of the utmost benefits of shifting into vegan is the improved level of health that you will undergo and this will show well beyond on your physique. In addition to this, the strong combination of healthy plant-based protein! The vegan diet is famous for its health benefits and especially for weight loss. Many people have made a vegan diet to lose weight and have succeeded.

Lose weight, enjoy more energy, and feel good by making a difference in vegetarianism. But before starting a vegan diet, you may be looking for a healthy and healthy diet to lose weight, and there are some things you should understand.

Most people make the mistake of giving the word 'diet' a negative connotation. It is for this reason that most of them are unable to stick to a diet when they want to switch to a different lifestyle. It is important that you do not do that. Tell yourself that you are switching to a healthier lifestyle that has numerous benefits. Remember that it is okay to give yourself one cheat meal. You can consume this meal on those days when you have cravings. You should remember to never make a habit out of it. Once you begin to lead a vegan lifestyle fully, you will no longer have any meat cravings.

Those who switch to a vegan diet get immediate benefits on their strength and note a better and faster muscle development. For an athlete also should not be underestimated the advantage of boosting the immune system, since it allows him to get sick less frequently and therefore, he can focus better on training.

Furthermore, in vegan nutrition there are no foods that are in fact pro-inflammatory, such as meat and dairy products, rich in cholesterol and saturated fats.

However, we should not make the mistake of believing that it suffices to be vegan so that everything goes well. Like any kind of nutrition, we need to make sure to incorporate a good variety of nutrient-rich food sources.

It is a good idea to structure a good personalized plan of weekly meals in order to be sure of assimilating everything the body needs. It is also good to feed several times a day and tossing away the famous rule of "three meals a day." High-end athletes eat up to 8-9 times a day, following their personalized nutritional program.

To be well prepared, the key is to have an unmistakable objective for the occasion, stick to individual plans and readiness procedures, remain at the time, and limit the effect of interruptions. Staying positive and hopeful, even despite misfortune, and overseeing feelings every day are extra tips that can have a major effect once rivalry shows up. For the groups who are set up for the experience, rivalries give energizing chances to exhibit capacities and are significant learning open doors for youthful athletes.

Now that you have learned the benefits of switching to a vegan lifestyle, and understand that there are ample plant-based or nut-based proteins that can help you provide your body with the necessary protein and other nutrients, it is time for you to get started with the reci